PALEO COOKIES

Gluten-Free Paleo Cookie Recipes for a Paleo Diet

John Chatham

ROCKRIDGE UNIVERSITY PRESS

CONTENTS

Chapter 3: Oatmeal Cookies

Chapter 4: Fruit Cookies

Chapter 5: Nut Cookies

INTRODUCTION

Cookies aren't just about delicious eating. They belong to cultural and familial traditions passed down from one generation to the next. Biting into a cookie can transport you back in time to your grandmother's kitchen or to those unforgettable family get-togethers of your childhood. In short, cookies aren't just a food: they're an inherent part of heart and hearth, which many find difficult to sacrifice in the name of health.

Until now, making the decision to eat healthfully has meant forfeiting many favorite foods, like baked goods traditionally made with nutrient-poor ingredients that do nothing but make you overweight and unwell. However, cookies are much more to us than junk food. For generations, cookies have held a special place in practically every culture. Americans have the chocolate chip cookie; Greeks create a delicious confection known as baklava; Italians munch rapturously on biscotti; and the British are renowned for their melt-in-your-mouth shortbread.

Thankfully, if you're one of those people who simply refuses to sacrifice tradition, eliminating cookies is no longer necessary. You just have to be willing to modify your recipes and experiment with some new flavors. This book will help you along the way. Traditional cookies are laden with all the bad stuff: white sugar, processed flour, and unhealthful fats. By replacing those bad ingredients with healthier alternatives, cookies can easily remain a part of your new, healthful lifestyle.

If you suffer from such conditions as diabetes, celiac disease, metabolic syndrome, obesity, or heart disease, leaving behind the Western diet is paramount to your health. Eliminating sugar, processed grains, gluten, and empty calories from your diet is a significant first step toward feeling better and living longer, but where should you start? From a clinical perspective, the Paleo diet is the perfect solution to managing your health issues, but from a realistic perspective, you may fear it's simply too restrictive to follow.

Throughout the following pages, you'll learn why it's so important to change the way you eat. You'll be introduced to healthier ingredients that taste delicious and open up a whole new world of flavors. As a matter of fact, once you try some of these recipes—including favorites like Paleo Chocolate Chip Cookies, Paleo Cutout Sugar Cookies, Chewy Paleo Coconut Cookies, and Paleo Lemon-Lavender Tea Cookies—you may find yourself more in love with cookies than ever before. Best of all, you won't feel guilty eating them!

SECTION ONE

Paleo Cookie Recipes

- **Chapter 1:** Chocolate Cookies

- **Chapter 2:** Sandwich Cookies

- **Chapter 3:** Oatmeal Cookies

- **Chapter 4:** Fruit Cookies

- **Chapter 5:** Nut Cookies

- **Chapter 6:** Holiday Favorites

- **Chapter 7:** Cookies with a Twist

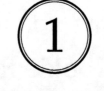

CHOCOLATE COOKIES

Paleo Chocolate Chip Cookies

Who doesn't love chocolate chip cookies? A popular favorite with just about everyone, they can be hard to give up if you're going Paleo. Lightly sweetened with maple syrup, these delicious cookies have less sugar than their traditional counterparts, but once you try one, you'll agree they are equally satisfying. Use the best-quality chocolate you can find for a true Paleo experience, as well as richer, better-tasting cookies.

- 3 tablespoons coconut oil, melted
- 2 tablespoons pure maple syrup or honey
- 2 teaspoons pure vanilla extract
- 1 tablespoon unsweetened almond milk
- 1 cup blanched almond flour
- 1/4 teaspoon sea salt
- 1/4 teaspoon baking soda
- 1/4 cup high-quality chocolate, chopped, or chocolate chips

---

Preheat oven to 350 degrees F.

In a medium bowl, and the coconut oil, maple syrup, vanilla, and almond milk, and beat to combine.

In a separate bowl, combine the almond flour, salt, and baking soda. Stir well.

Add the liquid and stir until well combined. Fold in the chocolate.

Line a baking sheet with parchment paper. Scoop rounded tablespoons of batter about 2 inches apart.

Bake for 9–10 minutes, until the tops are lightly browned. Remove from the oven and allow to cool for a few minutes before transferring to a wire rack.

Serve warm with a cold glass of almond milk.

Store any leftovers in an airtight container for up to 3 days.

Makes 1 dozen cookies.

Chocolate Hazelnut Meringue Cookies

These delightfully light and airy cookies have the same flavor as your favorite chocolate hazelnut spread, but without the refined sugar that accompanies it. While you can substitute maple syrup for honey in most recipes, stick to honey in this one, as maple syrup will overpower the chocolate and hazelnut flavors.

- 2 large egg whites
- 1/2 cup honey
- 1/4 teaspoon sea salt

- 1/4 cup hazelnuts, finely ground
- 1 tablespoon unsweetened cocoa powder

Preheat oven to 200 degrees F.

Fill the bottom of a medium saucepan with water, and bring to a simmer.

While the water is heating up, beat the egg whites, honey, and salt in a metal mixing bowl.

With the bowl over (but not touching) the water, continuously beat the egg white mixture until it is warm to the touch, about 5 minutes.

Remove the mixture from heat. Either in a stand mixer or with a hand mixer, beat the egg whites on high speed until glossy and thick, about 5 minutes.

Gently fold in the hazelnuts and cocoa powder, being careful not to deflate the meringue.

Line a baking sheet with parchment paper, and fill a pastry bag or a large Ziploc-type bag with the corner cut off with the meringue mixture. Carefully pipe the cookies onto the parchment.

Bake for about 90 minutes, until the cookies are dry and no longer shiny. Turn the oven off and leave the cookies inside for another hour.

Store in an airtight container for up to 1 week.

Makes about 2 dozen cookies.

Paleo Brownie Bites

While eating Paleo is generally a very satisfying diet, sometimes you just want to indulge in something rich and chocolaty without the refined sugar and grains that usually come along with it. This recipe for brownie bites will most definitely hit the spot. Full of dark chocolate flavor, these chewy, bite-sized treats are sure to become a favorite Paleo treat.

- 1/2 cup coconut flour
- 1/2 cup unsweetened cocoa powder
- 2 teaspoons baking soda
- 1 teaspoon sea salt
- 1/4 cup honey
- 4 large eggs
- 1 tablespoon coconut oil, melted
- 1 tablespoon pure vanilla extract

Preheat oven to 325 degrees F.

Combine the coconut flour, cocoa powder, baking soda, and salt in a large bowl. Set aside.

Add the honey, eggs, coconut oil, and vanilla in a medium bowl, and whisk until well combined.

Pour the egg mixture into the flour, and stir until well mixed. Allow the batter to rest for a few minutes. Stir again until the batter resembles a slightly thick brownie batter.

Drop the batter in rounded teaspoons onto a parchment-lined baking sheet about 1 inch apart. Bake for 8–10 minutes, until slightly puffy. Allow to cool completely.

Store any leftovers in an airtight container for up to 3 days.

Makes about 1 dozen cookies.

Paleo Double-Chocolate Cookies

Two kinds of chocolate make these rich and decadent cookies a treat you won't believe is actually Paleo friendly. While they are totally grain-free, you can make them vegan as well by replacing the butter with coconut oil. Since chocolate is the main flavor in these cookies, it's important to buy both high-quality cocoa powder and premium dark chocolate. Do this and you'll produce a deep, dark chocolate cookie that satisfies your chocolate cravings every time. In fact, these are sure to top your list of favorite Paleo treats.

- 2 cups blanched almond flour
- 2 tablespoons coconut flour
- 1/2 cup unsweetened cocoa powder
- 1 teaspoon sea salt
- 1 teaspoon baking soda
- 1 stick unsalted butter, melted
- 1/2 cup honey
- 2 ounces high-quality dark chocolate, chopped

Preheat oven to 350 degrees F.

In a large bowl, combine the almond flour, coconut flour, cocoa powder, salt, and baking soda. Stir until well combined.

Whisk the butter with the honey, and add it to the flour mixture. Stir well and fold in the chopped chocolate.

Drop the batter by rounded tablespoons on a parchment-lined baking sheet about 2 inches apart.

Bake for 10 minutes, until the cookies are dry and slightly puffy. Allow to cool completely before removing from the pan to avoid crumbling.

Store any leftovers in an airtight container for up to 3 days.

Makes about 3 dozen cookies.

Chocolate Shortbread Cookies

Intense chocolate flavor makes these cookies perfect for the Paleo chocoholic. With no other sweetener besides the sugar in the chocolate, these probably won't satisfy your sweet tooth, but you can easily add a tablespoon or two of honey if you'd like, or use semisweet chocolate instead of the bittersweet. Like anything made with chocolate, the higher the quality of chocolate, the better, and these cookies again prove the rule.

- 8 ounces bittersweet, dark chocolate, chopped
- 3 tablespoons unsalted butter
- 1/4 cup unsweetened cocoa powder
- 2 large eggs
- 1 tablespoon pure vanilla extract
- 1/4 teaspoon baking soda
- 1/4 teaspoon cream of tartar
- 1/4 teaspoon sea salt

Preheat oven to 375 degrees F.

Combine the chocolate and the butter in a large, microwave-safe bowl. Carefully melt the chocolate in the microwave, taking care not to overheat. Allow to cool for 5 minutes.

Once chocolate is cool, add the cocoa powder, followed by the eggs. Beat quickly until well combined, then add the vanilla, baking soda, cream of tartar, and salt.

Line a baking sheet with parchment paper, and spoon rounded tablespoons full of batter onto the cookie sheet about 2 inches apart. Use the palm of your hand or a spoon to flatten the cookies to about 1/4-inch thick.

Bake for 10 minutes and remove from oven. Allow to cool completely before serving.

Store any leftovers in an airtight container for up to 3 days.

Makes about 1 dozen cookies.

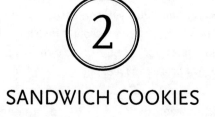

SANDWICH COOKIES

Paleo Whoopie Pies

Think you'll never eat a whoopie pie again now that you've embraced the Paleo way? Think again! These soft and chewy chocolate cookies have a creamy and delicious filling that will make you feel like you are breaking your diet, but you're not. OK, so you don't want to eat these every day, but for a once-in-a-while treat, they'll hit the spot every time!

For the cookies:

- 2 cups blanched almond flour
- 1/4 cup unsweetened cocoa powder
- 2 teaspoons baking soda
- 1/4 teaspoon sea salt
- 1/2 cup full-fat, canned coconut milk
- 2 large eggs
- 1/4 cup honey
- 1 tablespoon pure vanilla extract

For the filling:

- 3/4 cup palm shortening
- 3 tablespoons coconut oil
- 1 teaspoon pure vanilla extract
- 3 tablespoons honey

Make the cookies:
Preheat oven to 350 degrees F.

In a large bowl, combine the almond flour with the cocoa powder, baking soda, and salt, and stir well.

Beat the coconut milk with the eggs, honey, and vanilla extract.

Add the wet ingredients to the dry, and stir until well combined.

Line a large baking sheet with parchment paper, and use a 1/4-cup measuring cup to dollop evenly sized scoops onto the cookie sheet at least 3 inches apart.

Bake the cookies for 15 minutes, until the cookies are dry and shiny and lightly puffed up.

Make the filling:
While the cookies are baking, make the filling by beating all of the ingredients in a stand mixer. It will take about 5 minutes to beat until the filling is thick and creamy.

When the cookies are completely cool (and not a minute sooner!), spread some of the filling onto the bottom of 1 cookie and close it with the bottom of another. Eat right away.

Store filled leftover sandwich cookies in the refrigerator, although the filling will likely harden up a bit. To soften, simply microwave for a few seconds. Alternately, you can fill the cookies as you eat them.

Makes about 1 dozen sandwich cookies.

Chocolate Sandwich Cookies with Peppermint-Coconut Cream

Intense chocolate sandwich cookies filled with a cool and creamy mint filling? Yes, please! If you're looking for a special treat for a party or other gathering but want to keep it Paleo, you'll be head over heels for these chocolate beauties.

For the cookies:

- 1 cup blanched almond flour
- 1/4 cup unsweetened cocoa powder
- 1/4 teaspoon baking soda
- 1/4 teaspoon sea salt
- 1/4 cup coconut oil, melted
- 1/4 cup honey
- 1 tablespoon pure vanilla extract

For the peppermint-coconut cream filling:

- 3/4 cup palm shortening
- 3 tablespoons coconut oil
- 1 teaspoon pure peppermint extract
- 3 tablespoons honey

Make the cookies:

Preheat oven to 350 degrees F.

Combine the almond flour, cocoa powder, baking soda, and salt in a large bowl. Set aside.

In a separate bowl, combine the melted coconut oil, honey, and vanilla.

Add the wet ingredients to the dry, and stir until well combined.

Put the mixture into a pastry bag or large Ziploc-type bag with the corner cut off, and pipe approximately 1-inch rounds onto a parchment-lined baking sheet. Keep the cookies about 2 inches apart, as they will spread slightly.

Bake for about 8 minutes. Remove from oven and cool completely.

Make the peppermint-coconut cream filling:

While the cookies are baking, make the filling by beating all of the ingredients in a stand mixer. It will take about 5 minutes to beat until the filling is thick and creamy.

When the cookies are completely cool, spread some of the filling onto the bottom of 1 cookie and close it with the bottom of another. Eat right away.

Store filled leftover sandwich cookies in the refrigerator, although the filling will likely harden up a bit. To soften, simply microwave for a few seconds. Alternately, you can fill the cookies as you eat them.

Makes about 6 sandwich cookies.

Vanilla-Cream Sandwich Cookies

These lightly sweet cookies are slightly crisp on the outside and filled with a vanilla cream that makes them an elegant addition to a dinner party or other event. You can spice them up a bit by adding a taste of lemon zest, but they are simply delightful as they are.

For the cookies:

- 2 cups blanched almond flour
- 1/2 cup honey
- 1/2 teaspoon sea salt
- 6 tablespoons unsalted butter, softened
- 1 large egg

For the vanilla cream:

- 8 tablespoons unsalted butter, softened
- 1/4 teaspoon sea salt
- 1 cup honey
- 1 tablespoon pure vanilla extract

Make the cookies:

Preheat oven to 350 degrees F.

Beat all of the ingredients in a large mixing bowl until you have a thick dough. Wrap in plastic and freeze for about 10 minutes, until very firm.

Once the dough is firm, lay on a flat, clean surface and roll to about 1/8-inch thick. Using a 2-inch cookie cutter, cut out evenly sized circles and lay them on a parchment-lined baking sheet.

Bake for 8–10 minutes until the edges are lightly browned. Remove from oven and allow to cool completely.

Make the filling:

Beat the butter, salt, and honey in a mixing bowl until thick and creamy. Add the vanilla and continue beating until well combined.

Turn over the cooled cookies, place a small dollop of vanilla cream on one side, and top with another to make sandwiches. Enjoy immediately.

Store filled leftover sandwich cookies in the refrigerator, although the filling will likely harden up a bit. To soften, simply microwave for a few seconds. Alternately, you can fill the cookies as you eat them.

Makes about 1 dozen sandwich cookies.

Pumpkin Ice Cream Sandwich Cookies

When you've gone Paleo, you may assume you have to give up all kinds of foods, including decadent treats such as these amazing ice cream sandwich cookies. While these are definitely not an everyday indulgence, they actually don't stray too far from the Paleo principles. They're still filled with nutritious ingredients and contain none of the processed junk you normally find in treats like this.

For the cookies:

- 2 cups blanched almond flour
- 1 teaspoon sea salt
- 1 teaspoon baking soda
- 1 teaspoon cinnamon
- 1/2 teaspoon ground ginger
- 1/4 teaspoon ground nutmeg
- 1/2 cup pumpkin puree
- 1 ripe banana, mashed
- 1/4 cup pure maple syrup
- 1 teaspoon pure vanilla extract
- 1/4 cup coconut oil, melted

For the ice cream:

- 2 cups full-fat, canned coconut milk
- 1/2 cup pumpkin puree
- 1/4 cup pure maple syrup
- 1/2 teaspoon cinnamon
- 1/4 teaspoon ground ginger
- 1/8 teaspoon ground nutmeg

Make the cookies:

Preheat oven to 350 degrees F.

Combine the almond flour, salt, baking soda, cinnamon, ginger, and nutmeg in a small bowl. Stir to combine.

In a large bowl, mix the pumpkin, banana, maple syrup, and vanilla until well combined. Add the coconut oil and continue stirring. Add in the flour mix, and stir until well mixed.

Drop rounded tablespoons of the batter on a parchment-lined cookie sheet at least 3 inches apart, taking care to make sure they are uniform in size.

Bake for 20–25 minutes until golden brown. Allow to cool completely.

Make the ice cream filling:
Whisk the ingredients for the ice cream in a large bowl. Pour into your ice cream maker. Follow the instructions of your ice cream maker and freeze.

Once the ice cream is frozen, scoop even-sized scoops onto the cookies and sandwich together.

Store wrapped sandwich cookies in the freezer.

Makes about 6 sandwich cookies.

Lemon Sandwich Cookies

These soft lemon cookies contain a creamy lemon filling with a light, sweet flavor that is sure to delight your sweet tooth. For a twist, substitute the lemon with a lime or orange.

For the cookies:
- 1 cup blanched almond flour
- 1/4 teaspoon baking soda
- 1/4 teaspoon sea salt
- 1/4 cup coconut oil, melted
- 1/4 cup honey
- 1 tablespoon pure lemon extract
- 1 teaspoon lemon zest

For the lemon cream filling:
- 3/4 cup palm shortening
- 3 tablespoons unsalted butter, softened
- 1 teaspoon pure lemon extract
- 3 tablespoons honey

Make the cookies:

Preheat oven to 350 degrees F.

Combine the almond flour, baking soda, and salt in a large bowl. Set aside.

In a separate bowl, combine the melted coconut oil, honey, lemon extract, and zest.

Add the wet ingredients to the dry, and stir until well combined.

Put the mixture into a pastry bag or large Ziploc-type bag with the corner cut off, and pipe approximately 1-inch rounds onto a parchment-lined baking sheet. Keep the cookies about 2 inches apart, as they will spread slightly.

Bake for about 8 minutes. Remove from oven and cool completely.

Make the lemon cream filling:

While the cookies are baking, make the filling by beating all of the ingredients in a stand mixer. It will take about 5 minutes to beat until the filling is thick and creamy.

When the cookies are completely cool, spread some of the filling onto the bottom of 1 cookie and close it with the bottom of another. Eat right away.

Store filled leftover sandwich cookies in the refrigerator, although the filling will likely harden up a bit. To soften, simply microwave for a few seconds. Alternately, you can fill the cookies as you eat them.

Makes about 6 sandwich cookies.

OATMEAL COOKIES

Classic Paleo Oatmeal Cookies

While oats aren't a typical Paleo ingredient due to their being a grain, sometimes there's nothing better than a chewy oatmeal raisin cookie, and this recipe will fit the bill. Though the recipe does include oats, it does not contain any refined sugars or other processed ingredients you'll find in most other cookies. If you want something similar but without the oats, you can substitute shredded, unsweetened coconut, and you'll get a similar texture. One more note about oats: they are technically gluten free, but if you are following a strict gluten-free diet, make sure to buy oats packaged and labeled as such, since most common brands are processed in facilities with other products containing gluten.

- 1 cup blanched almond flour
- 1 cup rolled oats
- 2 teaspoons cinnamon
- 1/4 teaspoon ground nutmeg
- 1/2 teaspoon baking soda
- 1/2 teaspoon sea salt
- 2 cups full-fat, canned coconut milk
- 1/2 cup honey or pure maple syrup
- 1/2 cup raisins, optional
- 1/2 cup chopped nuts, optional

Preheat oven to 350 degrees F.

Combine the almond flour, oats, cinnamon, nutmeg, baking soda, and salt in a large bowl. Set aside.

In a medium saucepan, combine the coconut milk and honey or maple syrup. Bring to a boil while watching to make sure it doesn't boil over. Simmer for 10 minutes until nice and thick. Turn off the heat and allow to cool slightly, about 5 minutes.

Add the coconut milk to the dry ingredients, and stir well. Add in the raisins and walnuts, if you choose to include them, and mix well.

Scoop rounded tablespoons of the dough onto a parchment-lined baking sheet at least 2 inches apart and bake for 10 minutes or until cookies are lightly browned.

Allow to cool completely before serving.

Store any leftovers in an airtight container for up to 3 days.

Makes about 1 dozen cookies.

Nutty "Oatmeal" Cookies

These cookies don't actually contain any oats. Instead, they get their texture from a variety of nuts. Shredded coconut also helps mimic the texture of the oats so that you can omit them (they are a grain, after all). You'll love the pleasant taste and texture of these cookies and swear they could be Grandma's secret recipe.

- 3/4 cup coconut oil, melted
- 2/3 cup coconut sugar
- 1 large egg
- 1 teaspoon pure vanilla extract
- 1 1/2 cups blanched almond flour
- 1 teaspoon baking soda
- 1/2 teaspoon cream of tartar
- 1/2 teaspoon sea salt
- 2 tablespoons flaxseeds, ground
- 1/4 cup almonds, sliced
- 1/4 cup raw pecans
- 1/4 cup walnuts
- 1 tablespoon raw sunflower seeds
- 1/2 cup unsweetened coconut, shredded

Preheat oven to 350 degrees F.

Combine coconut oil, coconut sugar, egg, and vanilla extract in a small bowl.

Combine the almond flour, baking soda, cream of tartar, salt, and flaxseeds in another bowl, stir, and add to the wet mixture. Stir to combine.

Add the almonds, pecans, walnuts, and sunflower seeds to a food processor, and pulse until you have a coarse, sandy mixture. Add this and the coconut to the dough, and mix until well combined.

Drop by rounded tablespoons on a parchment-lined baking sheet at least 2 inches apart. Bake for 10 minutes or until lightly browned and slightly crisp. Cool before serving.

Store any leftovers in an airtight container for up to 3 days.

Makes about 2 dozen cookies.

"Oatmeal" Date Cookies

These grain-free cookies don't actually contain any oatmeal, but most folks won't be able to tell. Sweetened with dates and a little bit of honey, these chewy cookies are sure to be a hit with grown-ups and kids alike. If you don't have a huge sweet tooth, leave the honey out—the dates will do a fine job of providing ample sweetness, with the added benefit of some fiber and other nutrients as well.

- 10 dates, pitted and chopped
- 1 teaspoon cinnamon
- 1/4 teaspoon nutmeg
- 1 tablespoon coconut oil
- 1/2 cup pecans, chopped
- 2 tablespoons honey
- 1 cup unsweetened coconut, shredded
- 2 cups blanched almond flour
- 2 eggs

Preheat oven to 350 degrees F.

Put the dates, cinnamon, and nutmeg in a food processor. Pulse a few times, add the coconut oil, chopped pecans, honey, and coconut, and pulse again. Once you have a crumbly mixture, add the almond flour and eggs. Pulse until you have a rough, slightly wet dough.

Using your hands, form the dough into tight 2-inch dough balls, making sure to pack the dough well. Lay them on a parchment-lined baking sheet at least 3 inches apart.

Bake for about 15–20 minutes until the cookies are golden brown. Allow to cool completely.

Store any leftovers in an airtight container for up to 3 days.

Makes about 1 dozen cookies.

Oatmeal Cherry Chocolate Chip

These sweet, tart cookies do contain some oats, so if you want to go totally grain-free, even for a treat, you may want to skip these. That being said, they don't include refined sugars or flours, so they're not as bad as they could be. Tart, dried cherries and dark chocolate chips round out their delicious flavor, making them sure to be a favorite.

- 1 cup blanched almond flour
- 1 cup rolled oats
- 2 teaspoons cinnamon
- 1/4 teaspoon ground nutmeg
- 1/2 teaspoon baking soda
- 1/2 teaspoon sea salt
- 2 cups full-fat, canned coconut milk
- 1/2 cup honey
- 1/2 cup dried cherries
- 1/2 cup high-quality dark chocolate chips

Preheat oven to 350 degrees F.

Combine the almond flour, oats, cinnamon, nutmeg, baking soda, and salt in a large bowl. Set aside.

In a medium saucepan, combine the coconut milk and honey. Bring to a boil while watching to make sure it doesn't boil over. Simmer for 10 minutes until nice and thick. Turn off the heat and allow to cool slightly, about 5 minutes.

Add the coconut milk to the dry ingredients and stir well. Stir in the cherries and chocolate chips.

Scoop rounded tablespoons of the dough onto a parchment-lined baking sheet, at least 2 inches apart, and bake for 10 minutes or until cookies are lightly browned.

Allow to cool completely before serving.

Store any leftovers in an airtight container for up to 3 days.

Makes about 1 dozen cookies.

Spiced Oatmeal Macaroons

Without oatmeal, these are technically macaroons, but you'll be amazed at how much they taste just like your favorite oatmeal cookie. Egg whites make for a light and chewy cookie that is reminiscent of coconut and vanilla. Lightly spiced with cinnamon and ginger, they have a chewy, coconut-like flavor that is a cross between oatmeal cookies and coconut macaroons. Make sure you buy unsweetened coconut, as the sweetened varieties will make these overly sweet and difficult to enjoy the other flavors.

- 2 egg whites
- 1/4 teaspoon sea salt
- 1/4 cup coconut sugar
- 1 teaspoon pure vanilla extract
- 3/4 cup unsweetened coconut, shredded
- 3/4 cup almond flour
- 1 teaspoon cinnamon
- 1/2 teaspoon ground ginger

Preheat oven to 325 degrees F.

Beat the egg whites and salt in a mixer until you have soft peaks. Add in the coconut sugar and beat for another minute.

Stir in the vanilla and fold in the shredded coconut, almond flour, and spices.

Drop tablespoons of the mixture onto a parchment-lined baking sheet, about 2 inches apart.

Bake for about 12–13 minutes until the tops are lightly browned. Cool completely.

Store any leftovers in an airtight container for up to 3 days.

Makes about 1 dozen cookies.

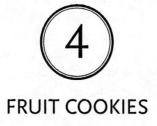

FRUIT COOKIES

Fruit and Coconut Breakfast Cookies

While eggs and other savory foods make up the bulk of Paleo breakfasts, sometimes you want something sweet and easy to grab. These cookies will fit the bill. Loaded with fruit and nuts, they are lightly sweet, full of fiber and protein, and can be eaten on the run. Feel free to substitute whatever dried fruit you like most to tailor these to your personal preferences.

- 2 ripened bananas, mashed
- 1/2 cup unsweetened applesauce, preferably homemade
- 2 tablespoons coconut oil, melted
- 3 pitted dates, roughly chopped
- 1/4 cup coconut flour
- 1 tablespoon cinnamon
- 1 teaspoon pure vanilla extract
- 1 teaspoon baking soda
- 1 tablespoon fresh lemon juice
- 1/2 cup unsweetened coconut flakes
- 4 dried apricots, chopped
- 2 tablespoons dried cherries
- 2 tablespoons golden raisins

Preheat oven to 350 degrees F.

Put the mashed bananas, applesauce, coconut oil, and dates in a food processor or high-powered blender, and puree until you have a thick paste.

Next, add the coconut flour, cinnamon, vanilla, baking soda, and lemon juice, and pulse a few times until combined.

Fold in the coconut flakes and the dried fruit. You can pulse once or twice if you'd like, but be careful not to puree the fruit.

Line a sheet pan or cookie sheet with parchment paper. Scoop rounded tablespoons of the dough onto the paper at least 2 inches apart, and flatten with the back of a spoon.

Bake for about 20 minutes, until the cookies are lightly browned. If you like crispy cookies, bake them longer. For a chewier cookie, bake for less time.

Allow the cookies to cool completely before eating.

Store any leftovers in an airtight container in the refrigerator for up to 1 week.

Makes about 1 dozen cookies.

Vanilla-Scented Apple-Cinnamon Cookies

These apple and cinnamon cookies are a delightful treat when you want something sweet but not too rich. Applesauce lends not only apple flavor but keeps them incredibly moist. If you can make homemade applesauce, these cookies will benefit from your efforts. Many apple cookies you'll find for the Paleo plan are filled with apples and dried fruit and are quite crunchy. These are the opposite: soft and moist, with a tender, comforting bite. If you enjoy other spices like ginger or nutmeg, they complement these cookies very nicely as well.

- 1/4 cup unsweetened applesauce
- 2 tablespoons pure maple syrup
- 2 teaspoons pure vanilla extract
- 1 tablespoons unsweetened almond milk
- 1 cup blanched almond flour
- 1 teaspoon cinnamon
- 1/4 teaspoon sea salt
- 1/4 teaspoon baking soda

Preheat oven to 350 degrees F.

In a medium bowl, combine the applesauce, maple syrup, vanilla, and almond milk. Beat to combine.

In a separate bowl, combine the almond flour, cinnamon, salt, and baking soda. Stir well.

Add the flour mixture to the liquid mixture and stir until well combined.

Line a baking sheet with parchment paper. Scoop rounded tablespoons of batter onto the paper about 2 inches apart.

Bake for 9–10 minutes, until the tops are lightly browned. Remove from the oven and allow to cool for a few minutes before transferring to a wire rack. Sprinkle the tops with more cinnamon if desired.

Store any leftovers in an airtight container for up to 3 days.

Makes about 1 dozen cookies.

Paleo Lemon-Lavender Tea Cookies

Just because you want something sweet doesn't mean it should be rich and heavy. Easy to assemble, these delightfully crisp cookies are bursting with lemon flavor and a hint of aromatic lavender. Real butter gives them a rich flavor that is perfect with a cup of coffee or tea. For variety, use orange or lime zest instead of the lemon, or if you prefer, leave out the lavender. Slightly crunchy, these cookies are sure to become a favorite afternoon snack.

- 1/4 cup unsalted butter, melted
- 1/4 cup honey
- Zest of 1 lemon
- 1 teaspoon dried lavender, crumbled
- 1/4 teaspoon baking soda
- 2 1/2 cups blanched almond flour

Preheat oven to 350 degrees F.

In a large bowl, combine the butter, honey, lemon zest, and lavender. Stir until well combined.

Add the baking soda and the flour, and stir until well combined.

Scoop the batter in rounded tablespoons onto a parchment-lined baking sheet about 2 inches apart. Lightly flatten with a spoon or the palm of your hand.

Bake for about 12–13 minutes until golden brown. Allow to cool completely before serving.

Store any leftovers in an airtight container for up to 3 days.

Makes about 2 dozen cookies.

Banana Bread Cookies

Moist and tender, these soft cookies will remind you of your favorite banana bread, but they are in fact grain-free and made with healthful ingredients instead of refined. Make sure your bananas are ripe enough; not only will they taste better but part of these cookies' moistness comes from the bananas—under-ripe ones simply won't cut it.

- 2 1/2 cups blanched almond flour
- 1 tablespoon coconut flour
- 1 teaspoon baking soda
- 1 teaspoon sea salt
- 1 teaspoon cinnamon
- 1/2 cup walnuts, chopped and toasted
- 1 stick unsalted butter, softened
- 1 cup pure maple syrup
- 2 large eggs
- 2 cups ripe bananas, mashed
- 3 tablespoons almond milk
- 1 tablespoon pure vanilla extract

Preheat oven to 350 degrees F.

Combine the almond flour, coconut flour, baking soda, salt, cinnamon, and walnuts in a large bowl. Stir and set aside.

In a mixing bowl, beat the butter with the maple syrup, and add the eggs, beating separately with each egg.

On low speed, add the bananas, followed by the almond milk and vanilla.

Add the flour mixture and beat on low until just combined.

Scoop the dough in rounded tablespoons onto a parchment-lined cookie sheet. Place them about 2 inches apart, as they will spread.

Bake for 15 minutes, or until the cookies are lightly browned. Cool completely before serving.

Store any leftovers in an airtight container for up to 3 days.

Makes about 1 dozen cookies.

Coconut-Blueberry Cookie Bars

These decadent blueberry bars are tart, sweet, and lightly scented with coconut. The dark color of the blueberries swirls through the coconut batter as it bakes, making for a lovely presentation. If you like, substitute whatever berries you have on hand; generally those in season make the best choice. Mixed berries make a great option here, too, so feel free to experiment with your favorite varieties.

- 1 cup coconut flour
- 1/2 cup unsweetened coconut, shredded
- 1 teaspoon cinnamon
- 1 teaspoon baking soda
- 1/2 teaspoon cream of tartar
- 1/2 teaspoon sea salt
- 1/4 cup honey
- 1 cup applesauce
- 2 large eggs
- 2 tablespoons coconut oil, melted
- 1 cup almond milk
- 1 cup fresh blueberries

Preheat oven to 350 degrees F.

Combine the coconut flour, coconut, cinnamon, baking soda, cream of tartar, and salt in a large bowl.

In a separate bowl, beat the honey, applesauce, eggs, coconut oil, and almond milk by hand with a whisk. Add in the flour mixture, and fold in the blueberries.

Brush an 8 x 8–inch baking dish with coconut oil. Pour the batter into the dish and tap lightly on the counter to settle.

Bake for 30–35 minutes until the top is dry and the edges are golden brown. Cool completely before cutting into 12 squares and serving.

Store any leftovers in an airtight container for up to 3 days.

Makes about 1 dozen bars.

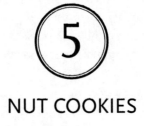

NUT COOKIES

Chewy Paleo Coconut Cookies

These chewy, coconut-flavored cookies are perfect for when you want something sweet but don't want to cheat on your Paleo diet. With the main ingredient being shredded coconut, they are full of chewy, toasted coconut flavor. When buying shredded coconut, make sure you buy the unsweetened variety; the standard, sweetened flakes you find in your store's baking aisle contain too much refined sugar to fit the Paleo diet. You'll find unsweetened coconut in the natural food section or a health food store.

- 1 large egg, beaten
- 3 tablespoons honey
- 1 teaspoon pure vanilla extract
- 1/4 teaspoon sea salt
- 2 cups unsweetened coconut flakes
- 1 tablespoon coconut flour

Preheat oven to 350 degrees F.

In a large bowl, mix the beaten egg with the honey, vanilla, and salt. Add the coconut flakes and mix until well combined. Add in the coconut flour.

Using a cookie scoop, scoop rounded balls onto a parchment-lined baking sheet, leaving 1 inch between each cookie.

Bake for 12 minutes, or until the cookies are browned and toasted. Cool completely before serving.

Store any leftovers in an airtight container for up to 3 days.

Makes about 1 dozen cookies.

Chewy Paleo Almond Cookies

This recipe contains only a few ingredients, but it produces delicious, flourless cookies both chewy and crispy at the same time. They also come together quickly, so these are a great option when you're expecting company and don't want to spend a lot of time in the kitchen. They're so chewy they almost resemble candy, and the slivered almonds toast up nicely to offer a satisfying crunch. Enjoy these with a cup of tea in the afternoon for a guilt-free pick-me-up. When baking, make sure you use parchment paper or a silicone baking mat, as these cookies are super thin and will stick to a baking sheet, even if it is greased.

- 2 large egg whites
- 1 cup sliced almonds
- 1/4 cup honey
- 1/2 teaspoon pure vanilla extract

Preheat oven to 350 degrees F.

Combine all of the ingredients in a large bowl and mix well. Line a baking sheet with parchment paper.

Spoon the mixture onto the parchment in round tablespoons. Spread the mixture into a flat circle, being careful not to make them too thin.

Bake for 20 minutes and check. If the edges are golden brown, remove them from the oven. If not, bake for another 3–4 minutes. Remove from oven and allow to cool for at least 15 minutes before removing from the parchment paper. Transfer to a wire rack.

Store cookies in an airtight container for up to 3 days.

Makes about 1 dozen cookies.

Paleo Chocolate Pecan Cookies

With rich chocolate flavor and crunchy pecans, you'll instantly fall in love with these beauties. Fairly quick to make, they are a great addition to offer guests or to add to a holiday cookie tray. You can substitute any chopped nut you like for the pecans; walnuts work particularly well, as do almonds. For a more unusual variation, try chopped pistachios; their vibrant green color and unique flavor will have everyone who tries them practically begging for the recipe!

- 2 cups blanched almond flour
- 2 tablespoons coconut flour
- 1/2 cup unsweetened cocoa powder
- 1 teaspoon sea salt
- 1 teaspoon baking soda
- 1 stick unsalted butter, melted
- 1/2 cup honey
- 1/2 cup pecans, coarsely chopped

Preheat oven to 350 degrees F.

In a large bowl, combine the almond flour, coconut flour, cocoa powder, salt, and baking soda. Stir until well combined.

Whisk the butter with the honey and add it to the flour mixture. Stir well. Fold in the chopped pecans.

Drop the batter by rounded teaspoons on a parchment-lined baking sheet about 2 inches apart.

Bake for 10 minutes, until the cookies are dry and slightly puffy. Allow to cool completely before removing from the pan to avoid crumbling.

Store any leftovers in an airtight container for up to 3 days.

Makes about 3 dozen cookies.

Mixed-Nut Maple Cookies

With four different types of raw nuts, these cookies are a nut lover's dream. They are slightly chewy on the inside but crisp on the outside and make a nice complement to a cup of coffee or tea. Feel free to add chocolate chips if you'd like, but you may find the addition overwhelms these multi-ingredient cookies.

- 3/4 cup coconut oil, melted
- 1/2 cup pure maple syrup
- 1 large egg
- 1 teaspoon pure almond extract
- 1 1/2 cups blanched almond flour
- 1 teaspoon baking soda
- 1/2 teaspoon cream of tartar
- 1/2 teaspoon sea salt
- 2 tablespoons ground flaxseeds
- 1/4 cup raw almonds
- 1/4 cup raw pecans
- 1/4 cup raw walnuts
- 1/4 cup raw pistachios, shelled
- 1/2 cup unsweetened coconut, shredded

Preheat oven to 350 degrees F.

Combine coconut oil, maple syrup, egg, and almond extract in a small bowl.

Combine the almond flour, baking soda, cream of tartar, salt, and flaxseeds in another bowl, stir, and add to the wet mixture. Stir to combine.

Add the almonds, pecans, walnuts, and pistachios to a food processor, and pulse until you have a coarse, sandy mixture. Add this and the coconut to the dough, and mix until well combined.

Drop by rounded tablespoons on a parchment-lined baking sheet about 2 inches apart. Bake for 10 minutes or until lightly browned and slightly crisp. Cool before serving.

Store any leftovers in an airtight container for up to 3 days.

Makes about 2 dozen cookies.

Pecan Shortbread

These sandy-textured pecan cookies are not terribly sweet, but they complement a cup of coffee beautifully. Lightly crisp, with the rich flavor of pecans, these are an easy addition to any holiday party or perfect pick-me-up to have around the house. You can substitute coconut oil for the butter if you'd like, but part of the appeal of these cookies is their rich and buttery flavor.

- 2 cups blanched almond flour, plus more for rolling
- 1 stick cold, unsalted butter, cut into pieces
- 1/2 cup pecans, finely chopped
- 1/4 cup honey
- 1 teaspoon sea salt

Preheat oven to 350 degrees F.

Put the almond flour and the butter pieces in the bowl of a food processor. Pulse until you have pea-sized pieces of butter. Add the chopped pecans and stir. Add the honey and salt. Pulse until you have a stiff dough.

Wrap the dough in plastic wrap and refrigerate for 30 minutes.

Lightly dust a clean, flat surface with almond flour. Remove the dough from the refrigerator and roll into 1/8-inch thickness, dividing the dough in half if necessary.

Using a 2-inch round cookie cutter, cut out cookies and lay them on a parchment-lined baking sheet about 2 inches apart.

Bake for 5–8 minutes, until lightly browned. Cool completely before serving.

Store any leftovers in an airtight container for up to 3 days. These cookies also freeze very well in an airtight freezer bag or other container.

Makes about 2 dozen cookies.

Almond Butter Cookies

Peanut butter cookies are a favorite among cookie lovers, but peanuts are a no-no on the Paleo diet plan. Luckily, there's a solution. With only three ingredients, these cookies are a great substitute for classic peanut butter cookies. They come together super fast—just seven minutes in the oven—leaving you with soft and chewy cookies but little mess. Take care not to overbake these, as they will firm up as they cool but taste best when they are soft and chewy. These are the perfect option when you want a healthful, homemade treat but don't want to spend hours in the kitchen mixing, baking, and cleaning. Make sure your almond butter is all natural, containing only one ingredient: almonds. Start to finish, these cookies are ready to serve in about ten minutes. How can you beat that?

- 1 cup smooth, natural almond butter
- 1 cup coconut sugar
- 1 egg

Preheat oven to 350 degrees F.

In a large mixing bowl, combine the almond butter, coconut sugar, and egg. Mix until smooth.

Line a cookie sheet with parchment paper. Drop the dough by rounded tablespoons on the cookie sheets about 2 inches apart.

Bake for about 7 minutes, being careful not to overbake. Allow to cool completely before serving.

Store any leftovers in an airtight container for up to 3 days.

Makes about 1 dozen cookies.

Vanilla-Almond Biscotti

Crispy and sweet, these classic biscotti are lightly flavored with vanilla for the perfect pairing to a cup of coffee or tea. They freeze really well, so make a batch and keep on hand for whenever you need an afternoon indulgence!

- 1 cup blanched almond flour
- 1/2 cup coconut flour
- 1 teaspoon baking soda
- 1/2 teaspoon sea salt
- 1 teaspoon pure vanilla extract
- 1/2 cup honey
- 1/2 cup almonds, sliced and toasted

Preheat oven to 350 degrees F.

In the bowl of a large food processor, combine both flours, baking soda, and salt. Pulse once or twice until thoroughly mixed.

Turn the machine on and carefully add in the vanilla and honey in a steady stream until you have a thick, stiff dough.

Fold in the almonds, but don't pulse the food processor or they will be chopped.

Line a large baking sheet with parchment paper and put the dough on top. Form dough into a log that's about 1 inch thick and 2 inches wide.

Bake for about 15 minutes. Remove from the oven and allow the log to cool completely before slicing. Don't throw away the parchment.

Once cool, slice into 1/2-inch-thick biscotti. Lay them on the same parchment-lined baking sheet and bake for 15 minutes.

For a softer cookie, remove from the oven, and cool on a wire rack. For a dryer, crisper cookie, leave on the baking sheet in a hot, opened (turned-off) oven until they are completely cool.

Store any leftovers in an airtight container for up to 1 week or more.

Makes about 1 dozen cookies.

HOLIDAY FAVORITES

Paleo Cutout Sugar Cookies

Looking for a way to enjoy holiday cutouts that fit into the Paleo diet plan? You've found them here. These few simple ingredients will produce cookies very close to those you know and love. Honey makes a great substitute for white sugar usually found in these cookies, but feel free to substitute maple syrup if you prefer that flavor instead.

- 2 cups blanched almond flour, plus more for rolling
- 1/4 teaspoon baking soda
- 1/4 teaspoon sea salt
- 1/4 cup honey
- 1 tablespoon pure vanilla extract

Preheat oven to 300 degrees F.

Combine all of the ingredients in a large bowl and stir to mix well. Using your hands, knead the mixture until you have a stiff dough.

Dust a clean, flat surface with almond flour. Using a rolling pin, roll the dough to about 1/4-inch thickness. You'll need to work quickly, as the dough will become much stickier the longer you wait to roll it out.

Using your favorite cookie cutters, cut the dough into shapes and lay them on a parchment-lined baking sheet.

Bake for 12 minutes and check for doneness. They are done when the edges are browned.

Allow to cool completely before icing.

Store any leftovers in an airtight container for up to 3 days.

Makes about 1 dozen cookies.

Paleo Gingerbread Cookies

Sticking to a Paleo plan can be difficult during the holidays, especially with all the temptations that pop up everywhere. Gingerbread is a traditional holiday favorite, and luckily you don't have to give it up. This recipe is easy to make and will give you the delicious, spicy flavor associated with these classic treats. If you need to take cookies to a holiday party but want to stick to the Paleo diet, bake a few extra batches; no one will know the difference!

- 1/2 cup molasses
- 1/4 cup pure maple syrup
- 3 tablespoons coconut oil
- 1 tablespoon full-fat, canned coconut milk
- 1/2 teaspoon baking soda
- 1/2 teaspoon cinnamon
- 1/2 teaspoon ground cloves
- 1/2 teaspoon ground ginger
- 1/2 teaspoon ground nutmeg
- 1/2 teaspoon sea salt
- 3 cups blanched almond flour

Preheat oven to 350 degrees F.

Put the molasses in a medium saucepan and bring to a boil over medium-high heat.

Once boiling, add the maple syrup, coconut oil, and coconut milk. Stir the ingredients until well combined and turn off the heat.

Combine the baking soda, cinnamon, cloves, ginger, nutmeg, and salt in a medium bowl and add the almond flour. Stir until well combined.

Pour the molasses mixture into the dry ingredients, and stir until well combined. Cover with plastic wrap and refrigerate the dough for 30 minutes.

Sprinkle some almond flour on a clean, dry surface, and remove the dough from the refrigerator. Roll out with a rolling pin until the dough is about 1/4-inch thick.

Using your favorite cookie cutters, cut the cookies into shapes and lay on a parchment-lined baking sheet.

Bake for 10 minutes until cookies are dry and slightly crisp. Don't overbake.

Allow to cool completely before decorating.

Store leftovers in an airtight container for up to 3 days.

Makes about 1 dozen cookies.

Paleo Pumpkin Cookies

Pumpkin is a nutritious vegetable full of vitamin A and beta-carotene. Unfortunately, when made into cookies, pumpkin can often turn into a diet disaster. With this Paleo-friendly recipe, you can enjoy your pumpkin cookies at Thanksgiving or other holiday parties without the guilt. Canned pumpkin works particularly well here, but you can also substitute mashed sweet potato or butternut squash for a unique version of these holiday delights.

- 1 cup blanched almond flour
- 1/2 cup pecans or walnuts, finely ground
- 1 teaspoon baking soda
- 1 teaspoon cinnamon
- 1/2 teaspoon sea salt
- 1 large egg
- 1 cup pumpkin puree
- 1/4 cup full-fat, canned coconut milk
- 3 tablespoons pure maple syrup

Preheat oven to 400 degrees F.

In a large mixing bowl, combine the almond flour, ground nuts, baking soda, cinnamon, and salt. Stir to combine.

In a small bowl, combine the egg, pumpkin, coconut milk, and maple syrup. Beat until well mixed.

Add the wet ingredients to the flour mixture and mix well.

Drop the batter by rounded tablespoons onto a parchment-lined baking sheet. Bake for 20 minutes or until slightly puffy and browned.

Store any leftovers in an airtight container for up to 3 days.

Makes about 1 dozen cookies.

Peppermint Meringues

These light and airy peppermint cookies are sure to be a hit at your next holiday celebration. While they take some time to make, keep in mind that the extra time is mostly hands off, while they bake and dry out in the oven. If you like, add a tablespoon of unsweetened cocoa powder along with the almonds for a chocolate peppermint cookie that is sure to please.

- 2 large egg whites
- 1/2 cup honey
- 1/4 teaspoon sea salt
- 1/4 cup finely ground almonds
- 1 teaspoon peppermint extract

Preheat oven to 200 degrees F.

Fill the bottom of a medium saucepan with water, and bring to a simmer.

While the water is heating up, beat the egg whites, honey, and salt in a metal mixing bowl.

With the bowl over (but not touching) the water, continuously beat the egg white mixture until it is warm to the touch, about 5 minutes.

Remove the mixture from heat. Either in a stand mixer or with a hand mixer, beat the egg whites on high speed until glossy and thick, about 5 minutes.

Gently fold in the almonds and add the peppermint extract, being careful not to deflate the meringue.

Line a baking sheet with parchment paper and fill a pastry bag or a large Ziploc-type bag with the corner cut off with the meringue mixture. Carefully pipe the cookies onto the parchment about 2 inches apart.

Bake for about 90 minutes, until the cookies are dry and no longer shiny. Turn the oven off and leave the cookies inside for another hour.

Store in an airtight container for up to 1 week.

Makes about 2 dozen cookies.

Classic Butter Cookies

Not all holiday cookies contain extravagant ingredients, and they don't have to be intricately decorated to be enjoyable, although you can certainly adorn these delicate butter cookies with your favorite holiday decorations. Real butter is the star of the show, and when sweetened with honey and vanilla, you have a deliciously flavored cookie that will be welcome at any holiday party. While maple syrup makes a fine substitute for honey in most Paleo cookie recipes, it would overpower the butter flavor here and leave you with a maple cookie. Unless a dominant maple flavor is what you want, stick to honey as your sweetener.

- 2 1/2 cups blanched almond flour, plus more for rolling
- 1 stick cold, unsalted butter, cut into pieces
- 1/4 cup honey
- 1 tablespoon pure vanilla extract
- 1 teaspoon sea salt

Preheat oven to 350 degrees F.

Put the almond flour and butter pieces in the bowl of a food processor. Pulse until you have pea-sized pieces of butter, then add the honey, vanilla, and salt. Pulse until you have a stiff dough.

Wrap the dough in plastic wrap, and refrigerate for 30 minutes.

Lightly dust a clean, flat surface with almond flour. Remove the dough from the refrigerator and roll into 1/8-inch thickness, dividing the dough in half if necessary.

Using a 2-inch round cooking cutter, cut out cookies and lay them on a parchment-lined baking sheet.

Bake for 5–8 minutes, until lightly browned. Cool completely before serving.

Store any leftovers in an airtight container for up to 3 days.

Makes about 2 dozen cookies.

COOKIES WITH A TWIST

Paleo Meringue Cookies

Light and airy, meringue cookies are an easy treat when you want something sweet. With only a few ingredients, you'll love these bite-sized delights. They are also simple to customize by adding extracts or other flavorings. If you prefer, maple syrup will work instead of the honey.

- 2 large egg whites
- 1/2 cup honey
- 1/4 teaspoon sea salt
- 1/4 cup almonds, finely ground

Preheat oven to 200 degrees F.

Fill the bottom of a medium saucepan with water, and bring to a simmer.

While the water is heating up, beat the egg whites, honey, and salt in a metal mixing bowl.

With the bowl over (but not touching) the water, continuously beat the egg white mixture until it is warm to the touch, about 5 minutes.

Remove the mixture from heat. Either in a stand mixer or with a hand mixer, beat the egg whites on high speed until glossy and thick, about 5 minutes.

Gently fold in the almonds, being careful not to deflate the meringue.

Line a baking sheet with parchment paper, and fill a pastry bag or a large Ziploc-type bag with the corner cut off with the meringue mixture. Carefully pipe the cookies onto the parchment about 2 inches apart.

Bake for about 90 minutes, until the cookies are dry and no longer shiny. Turn the oven off, and leave the cookies inside for another hour.

Store in an airtight container for up to 1 week.

Makes about 2 dozen cookies.

Maple Bacon Cookies

Although somewhat controversial in the Paleo world, bacon is a hot ingredient nowadays. If you've never thought of including it in a sweet treat, these delicious cookies will have you convinced in no time. When added to the batter, the crunchy, candied bacon offers the perfect balance of sweet and salty for an unusual treat that will have those who've tried it raving for more. Use the highest-quality bacon possible for best results.

For the candied bacon:

- 6 slices raw, nitrate-free bacon
- 1/4 cup pure maple syrup

For the cookies:

- 1/2 cup palm shortening
- 1/2 cup pure maple syrup
- 2 large eggs
- 1 teaspoon pure vanilla extract
- 3 cups blanched almond flour
- 1 teaspoon baking soda
- 1 teaspoon sea salt

Make the candied bacon:
Preheat oven to 350 degrees F.

Lay the bacon slices on a parchment-lined baking sheet. Drizzle the maple syrup evenly over the bacon.

Bake for 20 minutes. Remove from the oven, and allow to cool while you make the cookie dough.

Make the cookies:
Blend the palm shortening with the maple syrup in a large bowl. Add in the eggs and vanilla, and stir until well combined.

In a separate bowl, add the almond flour, baking soda, and salt.

Add the flour mixture to the wet ingredients, and stir until well combined.

Crumble the cooled, candied bacon, and add it to the cookie batter.

Drop the batter in rounded tablespoons on a parchment-lined cookie sheet about 2 inches apart. Bake for 13–14 minutes or until cookies are lightly browned. Cool completely before serving.

Store any leftovers in an airtight container for up to 3 days.

Makes about 2 dozen cookies.

Pumpkin Pecan Bars

Moist and tender pumpkin bars make an excellent choice for a fall treat, and pair nicely with apple cider or hot chocolate. Raw pecans sprinkled on top toast to perfection as they are baking, making your house smell delicious. Make sure they are raw, however—the long baking process will turn roasted nuts into burned nuts. Walnuts work in these bars equally as well.

- 1 cup blanched almond flour
- 1/2 cup unsweetened coconut, shredded
- 1 teaspoon cinnamon
- 1 teaspoon baking soda
- 1/2 teaspoon cream of tartar
- 1/2 teaspoon sea salt
- 1/4 cup pure maple syrup
- 1 cup pumpkin puree
- 2 large eggs
- 2 tablespoons coconut oil, melted
- 1 cup almond milk
- 1/2 cup raw pecans, chopped

Preheat oven to 350 degrees F.

Combine the almond flour, coconut, cinnamon, baking soda, cream of tartar, and salt in a large bowl.

In a separate bowl, beat the maple syrup, pumpkin, eggs, coconut oil, and almond milk by hand with a whisk. Add in the flour mixture and stir gently.

Brush an 8 x 8–inch baking dish with coconut oil. Pour the batter into the dish, and tap lightly on the counter to settle. Sprinkle the top with the raw pecans.

Bake for 30–35 minutes until the top is dry, the edges golden brown, and nuts lightly toasted. Cool completely before cutting and serving.

Store any leftovers in an airtight container for up to 3 days.

Makes about 1 dozen bars.

Key Lime Melt-Away Cookies

The same flavor as your favorite key lime pie, these sweet and tart bite-sized cookies are the perfect treat when you're dreaming of a tropical getaway. While regular limes will work in a pinch here, you should seriously consider seeking out key limes. They are slightly smaller, with a much more pronounced, tart flavor, and worth the trouble. Whatever you do, don't use bottled lime juice!

- 1 stick unsalted butter, softened
- 1/4 cup honey
- Zest of 4–5 key limes
- 2 tablespoons key lime juice
- 1 tablespoon pure vanilla extract
- 2 cups blanched almond flour
- 2 tablespoons arrowroot starch
- 1/4 teaspoon sea salt

Preheat oven to 350 degrees F.

Put the butter and the honey in a large mixing bowl, and beat on medium speed until fluffy and creamy.

Add the lime zest and juice, continue beating, then add the vanilla. Beat until very creamy.

Combine the almond flour, arrowroot, and salt in a medium bowl, and whisk. Add this mixture to the butter mixture. Beat on low speed until you have a stiff dough.

Divide the dough in half and roll into two logs, each about 1 1/2 inch in diameter. Roll these tightly in parchment or wax paper, and refrigerate for 30 minutes.

Remove the dough from the refrigerator. Using a sharp knife, slice the logs into cookies that are about 1/4-inch thick.

Lay sliced cookies on a parchment-lined sheet pan, about 1 inch or so apart. Bake for about 15 minutes until the cookies are very light golden brown.

Remove from oven and cool completely.

Store any leftovers in an airtight container for up to 3 days.

Makes about 3 dozen small cookies.

Green Tea Shortbread

You may think tea is only for drinking, while in fact it has many other uses, one of which is in these delightfully elegant, green tea shortbread cookies. Crispy and delicate, these cookies are sure to impress. Matcha is a finely powdered green tea that you can find at your local health food store or in Asian grocery stores. If you can't find it, simply grind some loose-leaf green tea in a coffee grinder as a suitable substitute.

- 12 tablespoons unsalted butter
- 1/2 cup honey
- 1/2 teaspoon almond extract
- 2 1/2 cups blanched almond flour
- 3 tablespoons matcha green tea powder
- 1/2 teaspoon sea salt

Preheat oven to 350 degrees F.

Put the butter and honey in a large mixing bowl and beat on medium speed until fluffy and creamy.

Add the almond extract. Beat until very creamy.

Combine the almond flour, matcha, and salt in a medium bowl, and whisk. Add this mixture to the butter mixture. Beat on low speed until you have a stiff dough.

Divide the dough in half and roll into 2 logs, each about 1 1/2 inch in diameter. Roll these tightly in parchment or wax paper and refrigerate for 30 minutes.

Remove the dough from the refrigerator. Using a sharp knife, slice the logs into cookies that are about 1/4 inch thick.

Lay sliced cookies on a parchment-lined sheet pan, about 1 inch or so apart. Bake for about 15 minutes until the cookies are very light golden brown.

Remove from oven and cool completely.

Store any leftovers in an airtight container for up to 3 days.

Makes about 1 dozen cookies.

No Sugar Added Cookies

These cookies contain no additional sweeteners—they get their lightly sweet flavor from a combination of dried fruit and coconut. These are a great choice when you have a craving for something crunchy but don't want to eat any additional sugar.

- 1 cup pureed pumpkin
- 1/2 cup unsweetened applesauce
- 2 tablespoons coconut oil, melted
- 3 pitted dates, roughly chopped
- 1/4 cup coconut flour
- 1 tablespoon cinnamon
- 1 teaspoon pure vanilla extract
- 1 teaspoon baking soda
- 1 tablespoon fresh lemon juice
- 1/2 cup unsweetened coconut flakes
- 4 dried plums, chopped
- 2 tablespoons dried cranberries
- 2 tablespoons almonds, finely chopped

Preheat oven to 350 degrees.

Put the pumpkin, applesauce, coconut oil, and dates in a food processor or high-powered blender, and puree until you have a thick puree.

Next, add the coconut flour, cinnamon, vanilla, baking soda, and lemon juice, and pulse a few times until combined.

Fold in the coconut flakes, dried fruit, and almonds. You can pulse once or twice if you'd like to bring the mixture together, but be careful not to puree the fruit.

Line a sheet pan or cookie sheet with parchment paper. Scoop rounded tablespoons of the dough onto the mat about 2 inches apart, and flatten with the back of a spoon.

Bake for about 20 minutes, until the cookies are lightly browned. If you like crispy cookies, bake them longer. For a chewier cookie, bake for less time.

Allow the cookies to cool completely before eating.

Store any leftovers in an airtight container in the refrigerator for up to 1 week.

Makes about 1 dozen cookies.

SECTION TWO

The Basics of the Paleo Diet

WHAT IS THE PALEO DIET?

Whether modern healthcare professionals want to admit it or not, the Paleo diet closely mirrors what most of them tell their patients: eat more fruits, vegetables, and lean meats, and stay away from processed garbage. The diet, also known as the Stone Age diet, the caveman diet, and the hunter-gatherer diet, has gained a significant following in recent years, and there's some pretty good research to support the switch.

How Did the Paleo Diet Start?

Back in the 1970s a gastroenterologist by the name of Walter L. Voegtlin observed that digestive diseases such as colitis, Crohn's disease, and irritable bowel syndrome were much more prevalent in people who followed a modern Western diet than they were in people's ancestors, whose diet consisted largely of vegetables, fruits, nuts, and lean meats. He began treating patients with these disorders by recommending diets low in carbohydrates and high in animal fats.

Unfortunately, the medical world simply wasn't ready to give up the idea that a low-fat, low-calorie diet was the healthiest way to eat, so

Dr. Voegtlin's observations and research went largely unnoticed, and the Paleo diet was shoved to the back of the drawer.

Finally—The Stone Age Is Cool Again!

Fast forward a decade to a point when medical researchers had gained considerably more insight into how the human body actually works. Melvin Konner, S. Boyd Eaton, and Marjorie Shostak of Emory University published a book called *The Paleolithic Prescription: A Program of Diet and Exercise and a Design for Living*, then followed it up with a second book, *The Stone-Age Health Programme: Diet and Exercise as Nature Intended*. The first book became the foundation for most of the modern versions of the Paleo diet, and the second backed it up with more research.

The main difference was that instead of eliminating any foods that people's ancestors wouldn't have had access to as Dr. Voegtlin did originally, Konner, Eaton, and Shostak encouraged eating foods that were nutritionally and proportionally similar to a traditional caveman diet. Because it was more realistic, the diet caught on like wildfire, and the research in favor of it continues to grow.

What Are the Rules?

Paleo is one of the easiest diets on the planet to follow: just remember to keep it real. If it's processed, artificial, or otherwise not directly from the earth, don't eat it. It's that simple. Here's a list of the delicious, healthful foods that the Paleo diet encourages:

- Eggs
- Healthful oils—olive and coconut are best; canola oil is under debate right now, too
- Lean animal proteins
- Nuts and seeds (note, however, that peanuts are NOT nuts)

- Organic fruits
- Organic vegetables
- Seafood, especially cold-water fish such as salmon and tuna in order to get the most omega-3 fatty acids

Sounds kind of familiar, doesn't it? That's because it's probably what your doctor encouraged you to eat more of the last time that you went to see him or her! Now let's take a look at some foods that are off the table if you're going to eat Stone Age style:

- Alcohol
- Artificial foods, such as preservatives and zero-calorie sweeteners
- Cereal grains, such as wheat, barley, hops, corn, oats, rye, and rice
- Dairy (though some followers allow dairy for the health benefits)
- Legumes (including peanuts)
- Processed foods, such as wheat flour and sugar
- Processed meats, such as bacon, deli meats, sausage, and canned meats
- Starchy vegetables (though these are currently under debate)

Frequently Asked Questions

Now that you have a general idea of what you can and can't eat, you may still have a few questions, so here's a list of those most frequently asked.

Q. Why do I have to quit drinking?

A. Beer is basically liquid grain, and it's packed with empty calories. Many types of alcoholic products contain gluten, which is discussed in detail in Chapter 10. Mixed drinks and wine are often loaded with sugar. If you absolutely can't go without that Friday-night cocktail, shoot for red wine, tequila, potato vodka, or white rum—and be careful what you mix it with.

Q. Why are legumes forbidden? They're natural foods and great sources of protein.

A. Most legumes, in their raw state, are toxic. They contain lectins—proteins that bind carbohydrates and have been shown to cause such autoimmune diseases as lupus and rheumatoid arthritis. The phytates in many legumes inhibit your absorption of critical minerals, and the protease inhibitors interfere with how your body breaks down protein.

Q. Why no dairy?

A. This one's under debate and there are many Paleo followers who still incorporate dairy regularly into their diets. The main reason that dairy is generally forbidden is that humans are the only animals who drink milk as adults, and many food allergies and digestive disorders are lactose related. There's a much more scientific answer for this question, but it boils down to believing or not believing that milk is bad for you.

Q. How will I lose weight eating fat?

A. This is a question that most people have initially because you're programmed to believe that red meat is bad for your heart. The fact is lean, organic, free-range meat is an excellent source of protein and many other vitamins and minerals. You're not going to be living on it alone; you're going to be incorporating it into a healthful diet.

Q. Peanuts are nuts and corn is a vegetable, so why are they off-limits?

A. *Au contraire.* Peanuts are legumes and corn is a grain. Be careful that you know what food groups everything you eat falls into or you may sabotage your efforts to be healthier.

9

THE BENEFITS OF PALEO

Many people turn to the Paleo diet because of the weight-loss benefits, but that's not where the idea originated. If you remember, the diet was created by a gastroenterologist to help his patients with various gastric disorders. Of course, weight loss is a wonderful side effect that has its own set of healthful benefits.

When you add in the myriad other perks, going caveman is almost a no-brainer. Let's take a quick peek at some of the biggest health benefits of following a Paleo diet.

Weight Loss

Since this is one of the primary reasons that many people decide to switch to a Paleo diet, this is a good place to start. Because you're eliminating empty carbs and adding in lots of healthful plant fiber and lean protein, losing weight will be much easier. A few other factors that contribute to healthful weight loss include:

- Plant fiber takes longer to digest, so you feel full longer.
- Lean proteins help keep your energy levels steady while you build muscle.

- Omega-3s help boost your metabolism and reduce body fat.
- You'll be eating a greater volume of food but taking in fewer calories.

The bottom line is that you'll be consuming foods that help your body function the way that it's supposed to, and one of the natural side effects of that is weight loss.

Healthy Digestive System

Remember that this was the original reason for the diet to be utilized. The theory is that people's bodies aren't adapted to eating grains, dairy, and other foods that are forbidden by the Paleo diet, and so they cause digestive upset, inflammation, and discomfort. Also, your digestive tract needs fiber to help it sweep food through your system or else it builds up and causes problems. Just some of the conditions that may be improved by going caveman include:

- Colitis
- Constipation
- Gas
- Heartburn
- Irritable bowel syndrome

Many people who begin the Paleo diet for other reasons, such as weight loss or heart health, report improved digestive health. Yet another reason that this incredible diet is worth your time!

Type 2 Diabetes Prevention

In the United States and other cultures that have adopted a Western diet, type 2 diabetes has reached disastrous proportions. Historically an adult disease, children are developing this debilitating illness at an alarming rate, and there's no sign of this trend changing. One of the main culprits is excess consumption of processed sugars and flours. By simply eliminating these calorie-laden, nutritionless foods from your diet, you can literally save your own life. The Paleo diet helps you avoid type 2 diabetes as well as metabolic syndrome, a precursor to many different diseases, for the following reasons:

- Omega-3s help reduce belly fat, an indicator of diabetes and metabolic syndrome.
- Lean proteins and plant fiber help increase insulin resistance so that your sugar levels don't spike.
- The vitamin C that's so readily available in citrus fruits and colorful veggies helps reduce belly fat.
- Lean protein takes longer to metabolize so you avoid energy highs and lows.

Immune Health

When you eat foods that your body isn't adapted to, such as processed grains, legumes, and dairy products, your body produces an allergic response in the form of inflammation, even if you don't experience any obvious outward symptoms. You may notice dark circles under your eyes as well as a feeling of general lethargy. You may attribute these symptoms to stress or exhaustion, but they're actually signs of a chronic allergy.

Inflammation in your body is a bad thing if it's occurring chronically, and it has been causally linked to such autoimmune disorders as:

- Fibromyalgia
- Lupus
- Multiple sclerosis
- Rheumatoid arthritis
- Several different types of cancer

The sad part here is that you don't even realize what you're doing to your body because there are often no symptoms until you have developed the disease. Switching to the Paleo diet may help reduce or eliminate your risk of many debilitating illnesses.

Cardiovascular Health

For most of your life, you've probably been told how horrible red meat and other animal proteins are for your heart, but recent research indicates that this is simply not true. Remember that there's a huge difference in scarfing down a fatty hamburger or sausage and enjoying a lean, organic, grass-fed steak. The burger and sausage are full of saturated fats and, most likely, hormones and additives.

On the other hand, steak is a lean, nutritious protein that delivers essential vitamins and minerals with very little bad fat and no empty calories, preservatives, or hormones. When you throw omega-3s and LDL-lowering healthful fats into the mix, you've got a heart-healthful meal that's good for anybody.

A Few Final Words on Health

The health benefits of giving up processed flour, refined sugar, and foods that cause inflammatory responses could fill an entire doctoral thesis, and the advantages to eliminating hormones and artificial additives from foods could fill another one. This chapter didn't even touch on how a Paleo diet can help with allergies, cancer, brain health, joint health, or celiac disease, but some of these will be covered in the discussion of the health risks of gluten in the next chapter. Suffice to say, the benefits of going Paleo far outweigh the relatively minor inconvenience of giving up a few foods.

THE TROUBLE WITH GLUTEN

Of the many health benefits of switching to a Paleo diet, one of the main benefits is that foods allowed on the diet don't have gluten in them. For millions of people worldwide, eating caveman-style is a relatively simple way to avoid digestive upset and even cancers that are caused by an allergy to gluten.

What Is Gluten?

Latin for "glue," gluten is a protein found in wheat and grains that gives the ground flours elasticity and helps them to rise. It's also the binding component that gives bread its chewy texture and keeps it from crumbling apart after baking. Because gluten is insoluble in water, it can be removed from flour, but typically when you do that, you lose all of the good properties that make breads and cakes what they are.

Without gluten, your baked goods won't rise and they'll have a grainy, crumbly texture. They won't taste anything like their gluten-laden cousins, and you probably won't want to eat more after the first bite. Because of an increasing demand for gluten-free products, food corporations have dedicated a tremendous amount of time and money into creating tasty, effective gluten-free products. Unfortunately, most commercially prepared gluten-free recipe mixes still fall short.

Is the Paleo Diet Gluten-Free?

Because gluten naturally occurs in wheat and grains, the Paleo diet is completely gluten-free. All grain products are strictly forbidden. Remember, the original creator of the diet was a gastroenterologist developing a plan that would help his patients with gastric disorders. Gluten intolerance is one of the most prevalent causes of gastrointestinal distress in Western civilization.

What Is Gluten Intolerance?

Gluten intolerance, or celiac disease in its advanced stage, is a condition that damages the small intestine, and it's triggered by eating foods that have gluten in them. Some of these foods include:

- Bread
- Cookies
- Just about any baked good
- Most flours, including white and wheat flours
- Pasta
- Pizza dough

Gluten triggers an immune response in the small intestine that causes damage to its inside. This can lead to an inability to absorb vital nutrients. Other illnesses associated with this disease include lactose intolerance, bone loss, several types of cancer, neurological complications, and malnutrition. Diseases notwithstanding, just the symptoms of gluten intolerance can disrupt daily life. They include:

- Depression
- Fatigue
- Joint pain
- Neuropathy
- Osteoporosis

- Rashes
- Severe diarrhea
- Stomach cramps

These are only a few of the symptoms that a person with gluten intolerance can suffer from, and since all foods that contain gluten are forbidden on the Paleo diet, you can see what the appeal is.

The Harmful Effects of Gluten

Gluten doesn't just harm people with fully developed celiac disease. It's actually harmful to us all. Long-term studies indicate that people who have even a mild sensitivity to gluten exhibit a significantly higher risk of death than people who do not. The worst part is that 99 percent of people with gluten sensitivity don't even know they have it. They attribute their symptoms to other conditions, such as stress or fatigue.

Absorption Malfunction

One of the attributes that many obese or overweight people share is the fact that they can still feel hungry after eating a full meal. This feeling of hunger is because gluten sensitivity is preventing your body from absorbing vital nutrients.

Food Addiction

There are chemicals called exorphins in some foods that cause you to crave food even when you're not hungry. Food addiction is a serious issue and doesn't necessarily denote a lack of willpower; these exorphins are actually a drug-like chemical released in your brain that creates an irresistible desire for more food. Gluten contains as many as fifteen different exorphins.

Though food companies have created gluten-free foods, they often replace the gluten with flavor-enhancers, such as sodium and sugar, which can still seriously sabotage your dieting and fitness efforts. Another advantage to the Paleo diet is that by following it, you're not only eliminating gluten, you're also avoiding the pitfalls of commercially prepared foods that continue to make you sick.

Other Conditions Related to Gluten

There are numerous other conditions related to gluten sensitivity, and many professionals postulate that this is simply because people's bodies aren't adapted to eating grains so they are treated as allergens. Other symptoms or disorders linked to eating gluten include:

- Anxiety
- Autism
- Dementia
- Migraines
- Mouth sores
- Schizophrenia
- Seizures

These aren't just minor aches and pains, though gluten sensitivity can cause those, too. These are major diseases and conditions that can ruin your life. It's no wonder that people who know that they suffer from gluten intolerance consider the Paleo diet.

Health Benefits of Going Gluten-Free

Obviously, there are countless benefits of giving up gluten, but here are a few that may be of particular interest to you:

- Decreased chance of several types of cancer

- Healthy, painless digestion
- Healthy skin
- Improved brain function
- Improved mood
- Reduced appetite
- Weight loss (or gain, if you're underweight because of malnutrition)

With the obvious advantages of giving up grains, it's difficult to understand exactly why people would hesitate. It's just a matter of making some adjustments to your diet, and now that understanding about both food and health is increasing, there are some great alternatives out there that will help you get rid of your addiction to grains!

(11)

PALEO FOOD GUIDE

S hopping for foods that are Paleo friendly can be a daunting task when you're first starting out. What's allowed and what's not? What are all of those mystery ingredients that are listed in foods? For the most part, stocking your fridge and pantry is fairly simple, but there are going to be times when you don't want to eat just steak and broccoli, and there will be other times when you need something fast and simple. Don't worry: you'll get the hang of it.

There are a few different versions of the Paleo diet, but this discussion will focus on the modern middle road so that it's easier for you to make the transition to your new, healthier lifestyle. Throughout the following paragraphs, you'll learn what foods are OK and where you can find them. You'll also learn some alternate ingredients for baking cookies and other goodies that won't get you kicked out of the cave!

Paleo Pantry and Kitchen Tips

The first bit of good news is that you're not going to be counting calories. Instead, you're going to try to keep your portions in line with what your ancestors most likely ate. A diet that consists of 50 to 60 percent protein,

30 to 45 percent healthful carbs, and 5 to 10 percent healthful vegetable fats, such as olive oil, avocados, nuts, and seeds, is the general goal.

Basically, when you're stacking your plate, put your protein on one side and your fruits and veggies on the other. Snacks can be whatever you want, but veggies and nuts are great choices. Be careful with nuts and fruits; though they're good for you, they're high in calories and can sabotage your weight-loss efforts if you're not careful.

If Possible, Go Raw

Many fruits and vegetables lose nutritional value when you cook them, so when possible, eat them raw. You'll also eat less because you'll be chewing more. If you opt to cook your veggies, steam them lightly so they maintain their bright colors. A key clue that you've cooked your greens to death is that they've lost that pretty vibrant green hue and turned an olive color. Try to avoid that.

Steaming, baking, grilling, and broiling are all great methods of cooking and require little added fat to prevent sticking. It should go without saying that the fryer can be retired to the garage to be sold at your next rummage sale.

Cooking on the Fly

Meals away from home can be a real challenge when you're first starting out. Restaurants are filled with tempting burgers and fries, and you have no idea what's in the salad dressings. If you must eat out, order a plain garden salad with oil and vinegar. You could also request a steak or chicken breast to go on top, but make sure that they either grill it dry or use olive oil.

Opt not to eat out in the beginning. Instead, make an amazing soup at home for dinner with enough leftover that you aren't tempted to go out for a quick fix. That way, you know what's in your food and you know that it's going to be delicious!

Plan Ahead

If you know in advance what you're going to eat for lunch or for dinner, you're not going to be as likely to cheat with something quick from the vending machine. Take snacks to work with you so that the box of doughnuts isn't so tempting.

Meats and Proteins

Your meats need to come from grass-fed, organic livestock, free-range poultry, or wild-caught fish and seafood. Wild game is great, too, if you're so inclined. Actually, meats such as venison are extremely low in bad fats and high in good fats and lean protein, so feel free to partake!

Fruits and Vegetables

If at all possible, shop at your local farmers' market for fresh organic fruits and veggies. Since the Paleo diet is dependent upon your creativity to complete a hot, fresh, delicious meal without the aid of flours, fats, and no-no's, you're going to have to learn a number of ways to prepare dishes. Plus, if you're offering a wide variety of foods that your family knows and loves, you won't be under so much pressure to create a single main dish that everybody will eat and enjoy.

Tomatoes are a great addition to any salad and make a flavorful base for soups and sauces. They're packed with nutrients and have so many uses that you should always have some on hand. Other staples should include carrots, peppers, cauliflower, and celery.

For fruits, opt for ones that are high in nutrients and relatively low in sugar, such as stone fruits and berries. Berries are also fabulous sources of antioxidants, phytonutrients, and vitamins. Apples are an easy grab-and-go food, as are peaches, oranges, and bananas. The dark tip of the banana that you usually pick off is rich in vitamin K, so eat it!

Oils and Fats

Oils high in saturated fats, such as corn oil and vegetable oil, are out. Opt instead for oils that are high in omega-3s, such as olive oil, avocado oil, coconut oil, and possibly canola oil. The latter is currently a point of contention among long-term Paleo followers, but there's a compelling argument to include it.

Seasonings

Your success with making the transition to the caveman way of eating is largely dependent on how flavorful your food is. As a result, you're going to need to incorporate various herbs and spices to make your dishes delicious. Here are a few that you should always have on hand:

- Allspice
- Black pepper
- Basil
- Cayenne pepper
- Cinnamon
- Cloves
- Crushed red pepper
- Curry powder
- Dry mustard
- Garlic—fresh and powdered
- Mustard seed
- Oregano
- Paprika

- Parsley
- Rosemary
- Thyme

Snacks

Finally, you'll probably want to keep some snacks on hand. Now, that does NOT mean cupcakes, potato chips, or crackers. However, there are still many options, such as certain beef jerky (or even better, make your own!), dried fruits, nuts, and seeds. They're satisfying and add nutrients to your diet instead of unhealthful fats.

Paleo Shopping Tips

Going to the grocery store is going to be a bit of a challenge at first, just as it is anytime that you make changes to your diet. Especially if you're accustomed to eating a large amount of refined flour and sugar and aren't yet over your sugar addiction, it's not going to be easy. Here are a few tips to help you along your way.

- Shop for your produce at the local farmers' market if possible.
- When at the grocery store, shop around the perimeter of the store. That's where most stores keep all of their meats and produce, and 99 percent of your food is going to come from those departments. If you need to get something from an aisle, go straight in, get it, and get back to the perimeter before those cookies catch your eye!
- Make a list and stick to it.
- If you do choose to eat canned fruits and veggies, make sure that you read the label so that you're not getting hidden sodium and preservatives.
- Buy meat in bulk when you catch a sale.
- Don't shop hungry! Have a low-fat, high-protein snack before you go so that you aren't tempted while you're there.

CONCLUSION

M aking the switch to a healthier diet can be daunting, especially if you've followed a traditional Western diet for most of your life. Leaving behind processed foods, unhealthful fats, and white sugar is going to require a true commitment, especially in the beginning, but if you're willing to push through that first month, you'll be amazed by how much better you look and feel.

You'll probably notice that your skin looks healthier, you've lost weight, and your energy level has doubled. Also, you'll feel full when you eat, and you won't crave sweets like a mad person, because if you've stuck to the Paleo diet, you no longer have a sugar addiction. That means that your cravings will dissipate nearly as fast as that spare tire around your middle!

Committing to the Paleo diet is often intimidating because of the many food restrictions; most people simply can't imagine life without sugar, flour, and all the tempting things you can make with them. Fortunately, now you don't have to. By using healthier alternatives such as almond flour, coconut oil, honey, and blackstrap molasses, you can occasionally enjoy sweets and treats that are actually good for you.

These recipes are just a springboard for your imagination—they demonstrate what is possible within the parameters of eating "caveman style." Now that you've got the hang of it and are in the Paleo frame of mind, you can experiment with your own favorite recipes, and continue your family traditions in a new, healthful way.

Unlike white flour and sugar, your new ingredients actually add flavor, texture, and dimension to your creations; you may just find that you enjoy the new, healthier versions you've discovered more than the old, fatty ones.

Good luck on your Paleo confections, and happy, healthful baking!

RESOURCES

Alternative Ingredients for Baking Paleo

Almond milk: Widely available in your grocer's dairy case, almond milk is a healthful, delicious replacement for dairy, consisting simply of ground almonds and filtered water. Characterized by an extremely mild, nutty flavor, almond milk is high in protein and low in bad fats. Unless stated otherwise, most brands contain added sweeteners, so be sure to buy unsweetened varieties.

Blanched almond flour: This is perhaps one of the most important ingredients in Paleo baking. While there are some other flours that are usable, blanched almond flour, in which the skins have been removed and the almonds ground to a fine flour, is hard to beat, and lends a mildly nutty flavor to your recipes. You can also make your own in a powerful blender or food processor by grinding almonds to flour, although it's difficult to know when to stop to avoid creating almond butter. Almond flour is high in protein and fiber and contains many more nutrients than refined, grain-based flours. Note that almond flour is different from almond meal, which is coarser in texture, and will not give you the best results when baking. Usually available at most grocery stores in the baking section; otherwise, check Amazon.com.

Cocoa powder: Unsweetened, natural cocoa powder. Available in grocery stores nationwide, but for higher-quality brands, check your local natural foods store or Amazon.com.

Coconut flour: Made from dried coconut that is ground into flour, coconut flour is extremely high in fiber and low in digestible carbs. Due to its high-fiber content, it's great as a weight-loss aid. However, coconut flour is rarely used as the sole flour for baking and should not be substituted for almond flour unless specifically stated. May not be available at your local grocer; check your local natural foods store or Amazon.com.

Coconut milk: You'll want to use canned, full-fat coconut milk in cookie recipes, unless otherwise noted. Coconut milk in a carton is made for drinking and is lightened up with water. In addition to its rich, sweet flavor, coconut milk boasts numerous health benefits, including maintenance of stable blood sugar and promotion of cardiovascular, bone, muscle, and nerve health. Often found in the Asian section of your grocery store. Native Forest makes a BPA-free version.

Coconut oil: An excellent butter substitute with a light but distinct coconut flavor. When purchasing, be sure to buy unrefined, virgin coconut oil. Coconut oil boasts a wide range of health benefits— good for your heart, your digestion, and your immune system, it is also useful in helping with weight loss. Melt in the microwave before measuring, and beware that mixing it with cold ingredients may cause it to seize up. Can be purchased at most grocery stores.

Coconut, shredded and unsweetened: Most shredded coconut you'll find in the baking section of your grocery store is sweetened with refined sugars, so make sure the package says unsweetened. May need to be purchased at a health food store.

Coconut sugar: Also known as palm sugar, coconut sugar is a sweetener made from coconut. You can find it at your local health food store or Amazon.com.

Extracts: When using flavorings and extracts, such as vanilla, almond, or lemon, make sure to buy only pure, natural extracts. Artificial versions have chemicals and additives that do not adhere to the Paleo diet. Most are available at your local grocer.

Honey: Pure, raw honey is the best sweetener for the recipes in this book. Be careful of flavored varieties, as the scent may come out in the final product. Locally produced honey purchased at farmer's markets or a natural foods store is best.

Leavening agents: Baking soda, baking powder, and cream of tartar are common items, although baking powder may be avoided in Paleo recipes, as it contains cornstarch. All of these are available in the baking aisle of your local grocery store.

Maple syrup: Always buy pure maple syrup, and make sure it states this on the container. National brands or any brands marked "pancake syrup" are simply maple-flavored, high-fructose corn syrup and should be avoided.

Palm shortening: A natural, vegetable-based, non-hydrogenated shortening that does not contain the trans fats of traditional versions. Great for replacing butter, it makes excellent frosting. May be available at your local grocer; otherwise, check your local health food store.

Salt: When using salt for Paleo baking, it's important to use a good sea salt instead of traditional table salt, which contains additives and preservatives. Keep in mind that even if you generally avoid salt, a small amount may be required for some leavening agents to work properly.

Sources/Brands

Amazon is a Web marketplace where you can find products of all types. Most of the items you need for this book can be found at Amazon.com, and sometimes for lower prices than you'll find locally.

Bob's Red Mill is an all-natural brand of gluten-free flours, shredded coconut, and other dried or powdered ingredients. You can find many of their products in your local grocery store's baking aisle, or at BobsRedMill.com.

Celtic Sea Salt is a maker of authentic, unprocessed sea salt, which will enhance the flavors of your baked goods. Go to CelticSeaSalt.com for more information on their products as well as where to buy.

Coconut Secrets makes a wide variety of all-natural products out of coconut. You'll find coconut flour, coconut oil, and other heart-healthful coconut products at CoconutSecret.com.

Penzeys is a nationwide retailer of high-quality spices and flavorings, including high-quality extracts and cocoa powder. Go to Penzeys.com for more information.

Spectrum is a brand of all-natural, organic oils available at grocers nationwide. Go to SpectrumOrganics.com for more information on their coconut oil, palm shortening, and other high-quality products.

Tropical Traditions is a maker of high-quality coconut products, such as oil or flour. Go to TropicalTraditions.com for more information.

Whole Foods Market is the world's largest natural foods store, with a variety of gluten-free and Paleo-friendly products. For locations, go to WholeFoodsMarket.com.

CPSIA information can be obtained at www.ICGtesting.com
Printed in the USA
LVOW08s0216091113

360221LV00003B/182/P